TESTOSTERONE DIET

The Ultimate Beginner's Testosterone Diet Guide & Action Plan - 30 Natural Fuelling Power Foods To Jumpstart Your Energy, Lose Fat and Increase Your Libido

By Freddie Masterson

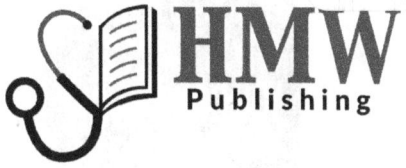

For more great books visit:

HMWPublishing.com

Get another book for Free

I want to thank you for purchasing this book and offer you another book (just as long and valuable as this book), "Health & Fitness Mistakes You Don't Know You're Making", completely free.

Visit the link below to signup and receive it:

www.hmwpublishing.com/gift

In this book, I will break down the most common health & fitness mistakes, you are probably committing right now, and I will reveal how you can easily get in the best shape of your life!

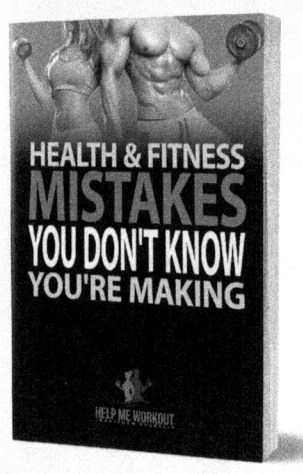

In addition to this valuable gift, you will also have an opportunity to get our new books for free, enter giveaways, and receive other valuable emails from me. Again, visit the link to sign up:

www.hmwpublishing.com/gift

TABLE OF CONTENTS

Introduction 8
    What is Testosterone? 10
    How the Body Creates the T-Hormone 10
        What is the Role of Testosterone in Males? 12
        What is the Role of T-Hormone in Females? .. 14
    The Level of Testosterone in the Body is Not Constant 15

Chapter 1 - The Marvellous Hormone, Testosterone 20
    What are the Normal Testosterone Levels? 20
        The Normal Range of Testosterone in Men 21
        The Normal Range of Testosterone in Women 22
    "Normal" T-hormone Levels Vary 22
    What Happens When the Body Has Too Much T-Hormone? 23
        High Testosterone in Females 23
        High Testosterone in Males 24

Chapter 2 - How Testosterone Benefits the Body and Affects Health 32
    Fights Depression 32
    Lose Body Fat 33
    Stimulate Muscle Growth and Mass 34
    Maintains Healthy Heart 36
    Keeps the Bones Strong 37
    Increase Sex Drive and Libido 38

Keeps the Mind Sharp 38

Chapter 3 - Signs Your Testosterone Level is Low 41

What are the Markers of Low Testosterone Levels 41

What are the Major Causes Low Testosterone Level? 42

    Aging 43

How to Treat Low Testosterone Level 51

    Hormone Replacement 51

Chapter 4 – Habits that Lowers Your Testosterone Level 56

Lack of Sufficient Sleep 56

Unmanaged Stress 57

Insufficient Dietary Fat Intake 58

Incorrect Dietary Intake 58

    Carbohydrates 59

    Protein 60

    Polyunsaturated Fat 60

Too Much Caffeine 60

Too Much Alcoholic Drink 61

Exposure to T-Lowering Chemicals 62

    Xenoestrogens 62

Foods that Kill Testosterone 63

    Soy-Based Food 63

Busting the Myth of Steroids and Drugs 64

    Fat Loss 64

    Muscle Growth and Strength 65

Chapter 5 – How to boost your testosterone naturally 70

- Get Enough Rest 70
- Relax 71
- Consume More Monounsaturated and Unsaturated fat 72
  - Monounsaturated Fat (MUFAs) 73
  - Saturated fatty-acids (SFAs) 73
  - MUFAs and SFAs Increases Testosterone Level 74
- Consume the Right Amount of Carbohydrate and Protein 75
  - How Much Should I Eat? 75
- Reduce Caffeine Intake 76
- Reduce Alcohol Consumption 77
- Avoid Xenoestrogens 77
- Hit the Gym 79
  - Lift Weights 79
  - High-Intensity Interval Training (HIIT) 80
  - Do Not Overtrain! 81
- Hit the Sack 81
- Take Cold Showers 82
- Bulk Up with These 83
  - 30 Foods that Boost testosterone Levels 84
  - Supplements that Aid Testosterone Production 94

Final Words 101

About the Co-Author 102

BOOK DESCRIPTION

Quit Feeling Sluggish and Naturally Boost Your Low Testosterone! Finally, learn about proven steps and strategies to boost your low testosterone. If you did not know, having low testosterone results in decrease muscle building, low libido (low sexual desire) and the feeling of being sluggish or lazy. However, there are natural ways to treat it and to boost your testosterone naturally!

This book will explain to you what this hormone does, what happens when it is found in low ratios in your body. How this hormone is working in your body. In what ways is it lowered, and will show you several natural ways to boost your it. This book will also make you discover how you can overcome your fear, and achieve heightened sex drive. If your sex life is disturbed or you are gaining weight without any possible reason, this book will be extremely valuable to you!

INTRODUCTION

When you hear the word testosterone mentioned, the first picture that comes to your mind are masculine men, working out, and body builders. You might also think of anger, aggression, or strength. You might even have a sudden flash of Arnold Schwarzenegger, and you would not be wrong.

Health experts regard it as the most significant male hormone. In fact, it is the ultimate male hormone. On the other hand, although the amount is considerably at lower levels, women also produce testosterone. Thus, although both sexes produce it, T-hormone levels cause more substantial effects on the male body and health than in the female.

T-hormone is the foundation of male existence, whether you like it or not. So knowing its importance and role, as well as giving it due attention is vital to your masculinity.

Also, before you get started, I recommend you **joining our email newsletter** to receive updates on any upcoming new book releases or promotions. You can sign-up for free, and as a bonus, you will receive a free gift. Our "*Health & Fitness Mistakes You Don't Know You're Making*" book! This book has been written to demystify, expose the top do's and don'ts and to finally equip you with the information you need to get in the best shape of your life. Due to the overwhelming amount of mis-information and lies told by magazines and self-proclaimed "gurus", it's becoming harder and harder to get reliable information to get in shape. As opposed to having to go through dozens of biased, unreliable and untrustworthy sources to get your health & fitness information. Everything you need to help you has been broken down in this book for you to easily follow and to immediately get results to achieve your desired fitness goals in the shortest amount of time.

Once again, to join our free email newsletter and to receive a free copy of this valuable book, please visit the link and signup now: www.hmwpublishing.com/gift

WHAT IS TESTOSTERONE?

T-hormones are the primary male sex hormone in men, and it belongs to a class called androgens, which you may know better as steroid hormones, natural or synthetic. Androgens are responsible for regulating the development of the maintenance of male characteristics.

Among the many androgen hormones, testosterone is the primary androgen hormone in males, which is vital for reproductive and sexual development. In fact, it is responsible for helping the body mature and prepares for sexual reproduction.

HOW THE BODY CREATES THE T-HORMONE

The endocrine system regulates the levels of T-hormone in the body. The production of testosterone begins in the cerebral cortex, the highly developed part that is often referred to as the gray matter and it encompasses about 2/3 of the whole brain mass.

The cerebral cortex signals two parts of the brain for the production of testosterone - the hypothalamus and the pituitary gland. The hypothalamus directs the pituitary gland how much testosterone to produce and the latter carries the instructions to the testes, with the communication occurring through hormones and chemicals in the bloodstream.

Specifically, the hypothalamus secretes gonadotrophin-releasing hormones (GnRH) - hormones that stimulate the release of testosterone in both males and females. The pituitary gland secretes luteinizing hormone (LH) and follicle-stimulating hormone (FSH), which travels via the bloodstream to the T-hormone producing parts of the body to stimulate the production and release of testosterone. This process is most active in the morning, and it starts to decline once there is sufficient supply of testosterone in the bloodstream, becoming less active at night.

What is the Role of Testosterone in Males?

In men, the testes are the primary producers of the T-hormone. Once the luteinizing hormone is in the bloodstream, the Leydig cells of the testes convert cholesterol into testosterone.

The adrenal glands atop the kidneys also make T-hormones, but only in small amounts. Specifically, the outer cortex or the outer layer of the adrenals produce androgens or family of male steroids, including testosterone. On the other hand, the medulla or the inner cores of the adrenals produce stress hormones, including cortisol and epinephrine.

In males, testosterone is responsible for many of the physical characteristics that are specific to adult men. It is the androgen involved in the development of sex organs before birth.

Specifically, this hormone is responsible for embryonic boys to develop male sex organs. After birth, it is responsible for turning a boy into a man during puberty, causing the sex organs to enlarge and become functional, as well as responsible for the following changes:

- Building and maintenance of muscle mass and strength

- Sperm production

- Growth of facial and body hair

- Lowering of voice

- Sex drive

- Penis, testes, and prostate gland enlargement

- Growth of Adam's apple

- Deepening of voice

- Broadening of the shoulders and ribcage

- Development of chin and jaw – the face remodeled and contoured

- Increase in height

- Changes in aggressive and sexual behavior

- Fat distribution

- Red cell production

What is the Role of T-Hormone in Females?

In women, the ovaries produce most of the testosterone, and the adrenals secrete it, too. In female bodies, the follicle-stimulating hormone from the hypothalamus stimulates the secretion of the luteinizing and follicle-stimulating hormones, which initiate the production of T in very limited amounts, mainly for reproduction. Although women produce significantly lower amounts, surprisingly, it plays a vital role for them as well, particularly in promoting the health of the following aspects:

- Muscle strength
- Bone density
- Sex drive
- Clitoris enlargement

However, when females have too much testosterone in their body, they cause male pattern baldness, along with irregular menstrual cycle, excessive hair growth, and development masculine body characteristics. Buzzkill!

THE LEVEL OF TESTOSTERONE IN THE BODY IS NOT CONSTANT

After puberty, when the body is sufficiently mature for reproduction, the endocrine system continuously produces testosterone, and the T-hormone levels are always changing.

Testosterone levels are at their highest in the morning and lowest in the evening. Often, various factors and conditions that affect the secretion of hormones cause the endocrine system to produce low levels of testosterone in the body. Uncommonly, the endocrine system instructs the body to create too much of T-hormone.

As mentioned earlier, the endocrine system controls the production of testosterone at the direction of the cerebral cortex, and this process is active in the morning. As the level of the hormone in your blood rises, the body will send a message to the brain, specifically to the hypothalamus, to suppress the secretion of gonadotrophin-releasing hormones. This process, in turn, stimulates the pituitary gland to suppress the luteinizing hormone production, which generally decreases the amount of T-hormone by night. However, several factors can affect the production and suppression of testosterone.

When the body is unable to stimulate and produce, as well as regulate and normalize testosterone levels – too little or too much - can create various health problems. Thus, it is vital to determine if your testosterone levels are well within the normal range. A simple blood test will determine if you have abnormal male hormone production. Once you have identified the status of T-hormone levels in your body, you can decide on the appropriate and suitable treatment to improve your hormonal problem efficiently.

Now that you know the role of testosterone on the various significant changes, as well as developments the body undergoes before and during puberty in both male and female, well will delve more in-depth about the importance of T-hormone. We will also tackle how age and various conditions affect the levels of testosterone and the other factors, as well as the personal habits that reduce the amount of testosterone secretion. Moreover, we will discuss what you can do to boost the production of T-hormone naturally.

If you suspect that your body is producing too little or too much T-hormone, go to the doctor and have yourself checked. Once you have officially determined the status of your testosterone level, you can begin stimulating and boosting or regulating and normalizing your T-hormones.

Key Takeaways:

- Testosterone belongs to a family of male sex hormones called androgens secreted and regulated by the endocrine system, primarily by the hypothalamus and the pituitary gland as directed by the cerebral cortex of the brain.

- The hypothalamus secretes the gonadotrophin-releasing hormone (GnRH) - hormones that stimulate the release of testosterone in both males and females. The pituitary gland secretes luteinizing hormone (LH) and follicle-stimulating hormone (FSH), which travels via the bloodstream to the T-hormone producing parts of the body to stimulate the production and release of testosterone.

- Once the luteinizing hormone is in the bloodstream, the Leydig cells of the testes convert cholesterol into testosterone.

- Testosterone is the ultimate male hormone. It is responsible for many of the physical characteristics that are specific to adult men.

- Testosterone secretion is most active in the morning, and it starts to decline once there is sufficient supply of testosterone in the bloodstream, becoming less active at night.

- The adrenal glands atop the kidneys also make T-hormones, but only in small amounts. Specifically, the outer cortex or the outer layer of the adrenals produce androgens or family of male steroids, including testosterone. On the other hand, the medulla or the inner cores of the adrenals produce stress hormones, including cortisol and epinephrine.

- Females also secrete testosterone, but in very limited amount and mainly for reproduction.

- When the body is unable to stimulate and produce, as well as regulate and normalize testosterone levels – too little or too much - can create various health problems. Thus, it is vital to determine if your testosterone levels are well within the normal range.

- A simple blood test will determine if you have abnormal production of the ultimate male hormone.

Chapter 1 - The Marvellous Hormone, Testosterone

The role of testosterone in human development in both male and female bodies is significant, particularly in helping prepare for reproduction and the physical traits of both men and women. In a very literal sense, the more testosterone is in a body, the more manly it becomes. So, what happens to the body when it has too much or too little T-hormone? Let us take a close look.

What are the Normal Testosterone Levels?

Determining the levels of testosterone in the body is a bit complicated. We distinguish the amount of T-hormone between *free testosterone* and *total testosterone*. What is the difference?

Well, a person can have high levels of *total testosterone* in the body but can have low levels of *free testosterone*. The latter is the amount of T-hormone that the body can readily use or disassociate from the proteins that carry them - albumin and sex hormone binding globulin.

A simple blood test can help determine the total, and the free testosterone levels in your body and the amount is often expressed in in nanograms (billionth of a gram) per deciliter [a tenth of a liter] (of blood), or ng/dL.

The Normal Range of Testosterone in Men

- Total Testosterone - 270 to 1070 ng/dL, with an average of about 679 ng/dL.

- Free Testosterone - 9 to 30 ng/dL, with an average of about 2 to 3% of total testosterone levels

The Normal Range of Testosterone in Women

- Total Testosterone - 15 to 70 ng/dL.

- Free Testosterone - 0.3 to 1.9 ng/dL, with an average of about 2 to 3% of total testosterone levels

"NORMAL" T-HORMONE LEVELS VARY

As you can see from the data above, the ranges of 'normal' amount of testosterone levels are quite broad. A T-hormone level that is within the healthy quantity for one person could mean hypogonadism (low testosterone levels) for another.

Hence, along with the actual *total* and *free* testosterone levels, you also need to consider the various symptoms you are experiencing when determining if you are well within your 'normal' T-hormone range or you have low amounts. For example, a middle-aged man could have no symptoms of low testosterone levels when the total amount of their T-hormone drops below 400 ng/dL, while a younger man could show signs of hypogonadism, which we will discuss further in Chapter 4.

WHAT HAPPENS WHEN THE BODY HAS TOO MUCH T-HORMONE?

Although less often than hypogonadism or low testosterone levels, the body produces high amounts of T-Hormones, and the effects depend on both sex and age.

High Testosterone in Females

We have mentioned earlier, testosterone is male sex hormones, and women only secrete only 10-20 percent the amount men produce. Too much T-hormone in a female can wreak havoc on a woman's body, mainly because their system is more sensitive to the levels of various hormones.

Excessive amounts of testosterone in a female body can cause deepening of the voice, increase in acne and body hair, and irregular menstrual cycle. High levels of male hormones, including testosterone, also cause infertility and polycystic ovarian syndrome, which can result in long-term health problems, such as heart disease and diabetes.

High Testosterone in Males

When boys have high testosterone levels, they can start puberty too early. In some rare conditions, certain types of tumors cause boys to secrete T-hormone earlier than usual. However, significantly high level of testosterone does not necessarily mean adverse effects in males. Higher than the average level of testosterone is actually beneficial, and even have positive results in men.

When your testosterone level is above 1000ng/dl., it means that you are in the top 2.5 percent of all males. It is interesting to note that men with above-average level of T-hormone display the following characteristics:

- Confident, assertive, and sociable
- Happier

- More energetic and have higher capacity for work
- Motivated and have greater ambition
- Healthy sex drive or libido, strong erection, quicker response time, and shorter rest period
- Increased concentration and have greater ability to complete complex mental tasks
- Great muscle mass increase and strength
- Lower body fat and higher resting metabolic rate
- Healthy heart
- Sharper mind

When is High Level of Testosterone Too Much?

However, excessively high testosterone levels have serious adverse effects to men's health, including enlarged prostate, hair loss, infertility, and acne on the shoulders and back, as well as the following signs and symptoms.

Low Sperm Count

Too much T-hormone overwhelms the reproductive system, causing reproductive problems. Sperm production decreases significantly, and can even halt until the body regulates and lowers the testosterone levels.

Shrinking Testicles

Excessively high levels of testosterone can completely shut down the testes activity, shrinking the testicles. If you notice a significant shrinkage of your testicular size, you need to consult your doctor right away. Men who undergo testosterone therapy of an extended period are prone to experience testicular shrinkage.

Mood Swings, Anger, Impulsivity, and Aggressiveness

Men with too much T-hormone can be happy one moment and furious or depressed the next. There is usually no trigger for this mood change, and any triggered emotion is overreactive. It is also harder for them to control emotions, especially anger, due to testosterone imbalance. They tend to act without thinking of the consequences first, and prone to hostility, usually acting overly aggressive. They often get into fights with other men.

Depression

Excessively high testosterone level disrupt hormonal imbalance, causing depression. Along with the loss of interest in activities they usually enjoy and sadness, a depressed person also experiences aching muscles, sleeping too long or insomnia, appetite loss, and weight fluctuation.

Prone to Addictive Habits

Research suggests that men with higher than the normal range of testosterone tend to smoke, consume alcoholic beverages, and participate in risk-taking behaviour, including injury risk, sexual, and even criminal activity.

How Often Should I Check My Testosterone Levels

One important thing to keep in mind when you are trying to raise the amount of your T-Hormone is that having higher testosterone levels for a long term can cause harm. To ensure that your level is within the healthy range, you have to start monitoring the amount every 5 years, beginning at the age of 35.

If your testosterone levels fall low or if you are experiencing the symptoms and signs of hypogonadism (see Chapter 4), you need to consider testosterone therapy. However, this remedy will require constant monitoring of your T-hormone levels, since excessively high amount can result in the adverse side effects mentioned above and stress.

If you have low testosterone level, the best way to stimulate and boost T-hormone production is by following the useful strategies we will discuss in Chapter 5. Moreover, finding the appropriate testosterone balance for you is possible when you consult with your doctor, as well as your willingness to check your T-hormone levels before initiating therapy and having it monitored routinely in the future.

Key Takeaways:

- Testosterone prepares the male and female bodies for reproduction and the development of physical traits in both sexes.

- The amount of T-hormone can be distinguished between *free testosterone* and *total testosterone*.

- A person can have high levels of *total testosterone* in the body but can have low levels of *free testosterone*.

- *Free testosterone* is the amount of T-hormone that the body can readily use, or the level that can disassociate from the proteins that carry them - albumin and sex hormone binding globulin.

- Total Testosterone in men ranges between 270 to 1070 ng/dL, with an average of about 679 ng/dL.

- Free Testosterone in men range between 9 to 30 ng/dL, with an average of about 2 to 3% of total testosterone levels

- The ranges of 'normal' amount of testosterone levels are quite broad. A T-hormone level that is within the healthy quantity for one person could mean hypogonadism (low testosterone levels) for another.

- Along with the actual total and free testosterone levels, you also need to consider the various symptoms you are experiencing when determining if you are well within your 'normal' T-hormone range or you have low amounts.

- When you are a man with testosterone level is above 1000ng/dl., you are in the top 2.5 percent of all males. It means you are manlier than most men.

- Excessively high testosterone levels have serious adverse effects on men's health.

- Men have to start monitoring the amount every 5 years, beginning at the age of 35 to ensure that their level is within the healthy range.

Chapter 2 - How Testosterone Benefits the Body and Affects Health

The hormones in our bodies are somewhat between remarkable and marvelous. There is a list of benefits you get from this which are astonishing and surprising. It is finally the understanding of how this hormone is more than the element of masculinity and is extremely useful and good for your health. There are several defects because of lowered testosterone levels; these are the benefits you will get because of them.

Fights Depression

The T- hormone helps fight depression. Studies show that men with low testosterone level exhibit more symptoms of depression. Furthermore, the research indicates that men with depression reported feeling much better and possess good mood after getting testosterone treatments.

LOSE BODY FAT

Men typically have less body fat than women do. Recent studies indicate that male hormones prevent the ability of specific fat cells to store lipids by blocking the signal pathway that supports adipocyte function or the storage of excess energy (glucose) as fat for more extended periods. Moreover, androgens increase the level of adrenaline (norepinephrine or epinephrine), which promotes the release of stored fat from its locations in the body, effectively helping you burn fat and increasing metabolism even during rested state.

The increase of adrenaline levels that allows the body to efficiently utilizes free and stored glucose (fat) in the body reduce the amount of circulating sugar in the bloodstream, which in turn, reduces the amount of insulin secretion. Insulin is the hormone that metabolizes glucose into energy.

In short, when you have low testosterone level, your body also has low adrenaline level. This condition means it has little ability to utilize fat and prevent fat build-up efficiently, which is terrible for your health. Excess fat is another reason to cause more decrease of the T-hormone level, fuelling the fire on the already precautions amount of androgens in your body.

Moreover, when the testosterone level declines, the estrogen level rises. It is the whole theory that explains why obese men or fat men have higher levels of estrogen and lower levels of testosterone.

Basically, all you need to do is to increase the amount of T-hormone in your body to break the evil cycle of having fats, and finally, become healthier. In another study, a person reported, he had lost weight, and his body fat had lowered from eighteen percent to twelve percent.

STIMULATE MUSCLE GROWTH AND MASS

When you ask gym goers how you can quickly build the muscle, as well as lose fat, they would probably tell you, "testosterone" or "steroids," and they would be right.

Androgens are the primary hormones that promote muscle growth. However, this relationship has to do with testosterone in relation to other hormones, specifically to adrenaline, insulin, and human growth hormone.

Growth hormone or somatotropin or human growth hormone (HGH or hGH) stimulates cell reproduction and regeneration and growth, thus, is very vital to human development. It is a natural hormone produced by the pituitary gland, and the majority of the secretion occurs during sleep.

As you age the level of HG production declines and it can lead to decreased lean muscle mass, lack of energy, and increase in body fat. Moreover, people with reduced HGH tend to have excessive body fat content. They also have reduced exercise tolerance and muscle strength.

You have learned earlier that high levels of testosterone increase the levels of adrenaline, which allows the body to utilize glucose as energy efficiency. In turn, this decreases the number of insulin levels in the blood. When the insulin level secretion decreases, it promotes the production of more human growth hormone (hGH), a hormone that efficiently burns fat.

Moreover, increase growth hormone levels in the body raise the amounts of circulating insulin-like growth factor I (IGF-I), which also regulate growth. The increase of both GHG and IGF-I results in the growth of muscle mass, as well as increase muscle strength.

Be sure to get you T-hormones checked out if you are contemplating on joining the gym to increase muscle mass and strength. Then follow the practical methods of raising your testosterone levels naturally in Chapter 5.

Maintains Healthy Heart

When we talk about the human body, the heart is of the highest importance, and there should be extra measures taken to assure its safety and its well-being. T-hormone also assists you with strengthening the muscle that pumps blood throughout the body and fight diseases. With ongoing researches, one of the studies tells us how testosterone helps with the cardiovascular disease, in a way that it strengthens your cardiovascular system, hence protecting you from it and cardiovascular system's related disorders.

KEEPS THE BONES STRONG

Bones gives us the idea that they are something that should be tough and well to process in the daily life chores. Testosterone also helps with making your bones strong. In older men, there is a very likely chance of getting osteoporosis, and as they grow old, the T-hormone also decreases. Hence old age mixed with low levels of T-hormone is not a good combination and makes your bones weaker. The process is simple; it goes as when the bone density intensifies, and it stops your bones to absorb the minerals, which forms poor bone absorption. So, be on your way to get treatments to increase the levels of testosterone.

INCREASE SEX DRIVE AND LIBIDO

The T-hormone is one hormone that is responsible for your sexual functions, drives or erections. So, if you are suffering decreased or low levels libido or sexual dysfunction, you know what to blame. Yes, it is the reduced level of testosterone that you can blame for your lowered erectile dysfunctions, sexual dysfunctions, and low libido. Notice the sharp decrease your sex life, make sure to check your T-hormone levels!

KEEPS THE MIND SHARP

Alzheimer's disease is one of the most feared diseases. Starting from your brain, your different parts of the body lose their function, you lose memory, or one side of your body loses its purpose. There is nothing scarier than that. Unfortunately, there is no direct treatment for it, but it slowly works out. What makes this better is the levels of testosterone in your body. Studies at the University of South

California and the University of Hong Kong reveal there are low levels of testosterone present in Alzheimer patients. T-hormone also helps with improving your cognitive impairment. Studies show a connection between T-hormone and cognitive impairment, which is also the case with memory loss. It also prevents brain tissue decay in elderlies. Competitiveness is one of the things that one always needs in different fields to secure their success. T-hormone also helps to increase the desire to win and to make one competitive.

T-hormones also increase your desire to have dominance and to gain power. And with it also helps woo a woman and also increase the risk-taking. So, all in all, make sure your testosterone levels are optimal.

Key Takeaways:

- Testosterone is not only responsible for turning a boy into a man and is also responsible for the male's health and well-being. A healthy and normal range of the ultimate male hormone level in the body fights depression, sheds excess body fat, stimulates muscle growth and mass, maintains a healthy heart, keeps the bones healthy, increases sex drive and libido, and keeps the mind sharp.

Chapter 3 - Signs Your Testosterone Level is Low

A low T-hormone level is the most common out of normal range for in men. How do you know if your male hormone is below the healthy amount? Here are the markers and the most common symptoms.

What are the Markers of Low Testosterone Levels

When T-hormones cannot separate from the protein carriers albumin and the sex hormone binding globulin, they are not readily available for use by the body, which results in the symptoms of low T-hormone levels or hypogonadism.

A research pointed out that men younger than 40 years old could have symptoms low testosterone levels when the total amount of their T-hormone drops below 400 ng/dL.

On the other hand, a study revealed that mean between 40 to 90 years old show symptoms low testosterone levels when the when the total amount of their T-hormone drops below 300 ng/dL.

Moreover, some research suggests that the healthiest men have testosterone levels between 400 to 600 ng/dL, which gives you an idea if you re within the 'normal' range.

So if your testosterone levels are below the markers for your age group or if you are experiencing the signs and hypogonadism symptoms, then you need to confirm your suspicion by doing a blood test.

What are the Major Causes Low Testosterone Level?

It is easy to discover your T-levels are lower than average by doing blood tests, but what might be the reason behind it?

Aging

As mentioned earlier, the normal range of male T-hormone level is about 270 to 1070 ng/dL with an average level of 679 ng/dL. Your testosterone level is at its peak when you are around 20 years old, and then it slowly starts to decline. Research suggests that each year T-hormone level decrease by 1 percent in middle-aged males between 30 to 50 years old and older men.

The decline may be noticeable in some males, and others may experience noticeable changes beginning in their middle-age years or more commonly when they are around 60 years old and older.

You may have heard the terms andropause or "male menopause," the name given to describe the drop in male T-hormone level. This is what most health experts refer to as hypogonadism.

Testicular Failure

As mentioned earlier, the primary producers of T-hormone in males are the testes. The primary cause of hypogonadism is a testicular failure, which can be due to sex hormones congenital abnormality, including the following conditions:

- Klinefelter's syndrome results in testosterone underproduction due to the extra X chromosome added to the XY of a healthy male.

- Mump infection affecting the testicles experienced with mumps of the salivary gland occurring during adulthood or adolescence can cause long-term damage to the testes.

- Hemochromatosis or too much amount of iron in the blood can cause pituitary gland or testicular dysfunction or failure.

- Injury to your testicles can cause hypogonadism since they are located outside the body, making them prone to damage and injury.

- Testicular cancer lowers testosterone levels so get yourself checked.

- Cancer treatment can inhibit with sperm and testosterone production, which can lead to temporary or permanent infertility.

Hypothalamus or Pituitary Problems

Problems involving the hypothalamus or pituitary are the secondary cause of hypogonadism. As mentioned earlier, these two parts of the brain regulate the production of testosterone in the testes.

Secondary hypogonadism is often due to the following causes:

- Kallmann syndrome results in abnormal hypothalamus development, also associated with anosmia or impaired ability to smell, affects the secretion of pituitary hormones.

- Pituitary disorders impair hormone release to the testicles, resulting in abnormal T-hormone production, and this can include pituitary or other brain tumors, as well as treatment.

- Inflammatory disease, such as tuberculosis, Histiocytosis, and sarcoidosis involves the hypothalamus and pituitary gland, causing hypogonadism.

- HIV/AIDS affects the hypothalamus and pituitary, as well as the testes.

- Medications and certain hormones affect T-hormone production.

- Stress, weight loss, and excessive physical activity can cause hypogonadism.

- Head trauma can also affect T-hormone level since the pituitary gland regulates the production of the male hormone.

Other factors may include chronic liver, kidney disease, Type 2 diabetes, or obesity.

The Hypogonadism Symptoms in Men and Women

Some of the signs are mistaken for old age symptoms, or sometimes you are too busy to care about what is happening in your body. But, all the signs and warnings for hypogonadism that you should carefully look into are the following:

General Symptoms

- Lessened sex drive
- Erectile brokenness or ineptitude
- Expanded breast size
- Brought down sperm tally
- Hot flashes
- Depression, irritability, and failure to think
- Contracted and relaxed testes

- Loss of bulk or hair

- Bones getting to be inclined to break

For starters, you feel less energetic and fatigue filling your entire body. You feel sleepier than usual. Anyone can be sluggish or lazy to go to the gym, or even you are entirely up to it, you think you are not running on the treadmill as before. Which brings low self-esteem issues, and you end up sitting at home. The motivation you had started to hit the gym is gone. Despite sleeping more than usual, you still feel lethargic, in any of these cases; make sure to get your T-levels checked.

Then, your sex drive declines, the T-hormone works in the sex drive same with both men and women. If your sex drives are low, or you do not feel too much sexually active, make sure to get your T-levels checked. In women, the hormonal changes will also make sure the changes in mood and might influence mood swings.

As mentioned earlier, T-hormone helps with gaining muscle mass; it works opposite as well. If you feel in the slightest, any change in your muscle mass, be sure to check it because once it is at a loss, it is hard to rebuild.

Another sign is your low semen quantity. So basically, if you feel less sperm production or less sperm in an ejaculation, make sure to get your testosterone levels checked.

One of the most infuriating problems is hair loss. The amount of hair products you get or the amount of time you put oil on your hair is hectic. Facial hair is one of the things a man is proud of; there is nothing sadder than losing your beard's thick hair. Balding is natural for old age, but if you are shedding facial and body hair, you lack in the T-hormone levels.

One of the other warnings you might get from your body is the lower bone mass. As mentioned earlier, it helps to prevent osteoporosis and prevents thinning of the bones.

Another of the side effects, you might feel significant mood problems.

Ladies regularly encounter changes in mindset amid menopause when levels of estrogen drop. Men with lesser T can experience comparable manifestations. Testosterone affects various physical methods in the body.

The more specific symptoms of low testosterone levels in men and women are the following.

Hypogonadism Symptoms in Males

- Loss of body hair
- Muscle damage
- Unusual breast development
- Decreased growth of penis and testicles
- Erectile dysfunction
- Osteoporosis
- Less or missing sex drive
- Infertility
- Weariness
- Hot flashes
- Trouble concentrating

Hypogonadism Symptoms in Females

- Absence of feminine cycle
- Moderate or missing breast development
- Hot flashes
- Loss of body hair
- Low or missing sex drive
- Milky release from your breasts

HOW TO TREAT LOW TESTOSTERONE LEVEL

Testosterone treatment is the most common remedy for male hypogonadism. The correct one will depend on the cause, as well as concerns about fertility. The most common involve the following:

Hormone Replacement

Testosterone replacement therapy (TRT) in boys help stimulate puberty and development, including penile and testicle growth, pubic hair and beard growth, and muscle mass increase. TRT for boys often include the following methods:

- Testosterone enanthate, testosterone cypionate, and testosterone undecanoate (Aveed) injection
- in the muscle.
- Patch applied every night on the thigh, upper arm, abdomen, or back.
- Gel rubbed on the shoulder or upper arm, under each armpit, or on the inner or front thigh.
- A putty-like substance placed where the upper lip meets the gum or the buccal cavity.
- Gels pumped into each nostril 2 to 3 times a day.
- Implantable pellets that are surgically placed under the skin every 3 to 6 months.

In men, TRT helps restore muscle strength and prevent bone loss. Men receiving treatment also experience increased erectile function, sex drive, energy, and sense of well-being. It also restores fertility and stimulates sperm production.

However, it is only used when fertility is not the issue. For men who have been unsuccessful in achieving conception with their partner, assisted reproductive technology may be helpful. Assisted reproduction covers a wide array of techniques designed to help couples conceive.

However, testosterone replacement therapy carries various risks, including the following:

- Blood clots formation in the veins

- Stimulate the growth of pre-existing prostate cancer

- Limit sperm production

- Breast enlargement

- Stimulating noncancerous prostate growth

- Sleep Apnea

- Increase risk of heart attack

Thus, stimulating the production of testosterone level the natural way is the best solution for hypogonadism.

Key Takeaways:

- Men younger than 40 years old could have symptoms low testosterone levels when the total amount of their T-hormone drops below 400 ng/dL.

- Men between 40 to 90 years old show symptoms low testosterone levels when the when the total amount of their T-hormone drops below 300 ng/dL.

- The healthiest men have testosterone levels between 400 to 600 ng/dL, what we refer to as the 'normal' range.

- Aging is the number one cause of low testosterone level.

- Testosterone level is at its peak when you are around 20 years old, and then it slowly starts to decline.

- Each year, T-hormone level decrease by 1 percent in middle-aged males between 30 to 50 years old and older men.

- Testicular failure is the primary cause of andropause or "male menopause."

- Problems involving the hypothalamus or pituitary are the secondary cause of hypogonadism.

- In men, hypogonadism symptoms include loss of body hair, muscle damage, unusual breast development, decreased growth of penis and testicles, erectile dysfunction. Osteoporosis, less or missing sex drive, infertility, weariness, hot flashes, and trouble concentrating.

- Hypogonadism can be treated with testosterone replacement therapy (TRT), but this solution carries specific risks, including blood clots formation in the veins, stimulate the growth of pre-existing prostate cancer, limit sperm production, breast enlargement, encouraging noncancerous prostate growth, sleep apnea, and increase the risk of heart attack.

Chapter 4 – Habits that Lowers Your Testosterone Level

Aside from the natural causes of testosterone decline, aging, testicular failure, and hypothalamus or pituitary problems, your lifestyle dramatically influences the production of the male hormone. What habits sabotage your manliness?

Lack of Sufficient Sleep

Most people today do not get enough sleep, which is one of the primary factors that affect the production of testosterone in males. Studies reveal that the body makes almost all the T it needs for the day during sleeping. The increased level of testosterone at night is one of the main reasons why men wake up with "morning wood." In fact, consistently waking up "hard" means you have a healthy amount of the male hormone.

If you are sleep deprived, your body cannot produce T as effectively or efficiently. A study revealed that young men who are fully rested had higher T-hormone levels than those who sleep less than 5 hours every night for 1 week. The amount of testosterone of men who lack sufficient rest dropped around 10 to 15 percent.

Enough sleep also helps regulate cortisol, a stress hormone that reduces blood T-hormone level when in high amounts. Getting enough rest when you experience any form of stress is specifically vital because it increases the cortisol level significantly, which disrupts T production.

UNMANAGED STRESS

Short-term and chronic long-term stress hammer T-hormone production in two ways. First, psychological and physical stress stimulates increased secretion of cortisol from the adrenal cortex, which suppresses the role of the hypothalamus and testes in T-hormone production.

Secondly, cortisol synthesis requires cholesterol, a molecule that is also vital in testosterone biosynthesis. When stress hormones skyrocket, the body utilizes cholesterol more for creating cortisol than T-hormone.

INSUFFICIENT DIETARY FAT INTAKE

Your body's ability to produce male hormone efficiently depends significantly on your dietary fat intake. Fat contains cholesterol. As mentioned earlier, this molecule is vital to testosterone production.

In fact, cholesterol from fat converts to steroidal hormones, testosterone, and estrogen as well. Consuming less than 20 percent of calories from fat will limit your testosterone production. Eating enough HEALTHY fats is vital to maintaining not just T, but other hormone production.

INCORRECT DIETARY INTAKE

Your nutritional intake influences male hormone production significantly. As mentioned earlier, your testosterone level dramatically depends on the active or free T-hormone in the blood, the ones that your body can readily utilize.

Active or free testosterone in your blood travels to your muscle cells and other tissues. In some tissues, such as brain and fat cells, your body could covert fat into the female hormone estrogen depending on your nutrient intake. When your diet stimulates excessive production of estrogen, it can lead to fat gain, which further inhibits T production by decreasing brain hormones.

Carbohydrates

As mentioned earlier, the body needs adequate amounts of calories for testosterone production. Consuming insufficient amount of calorie from carbs reduces messenger hormones secreted by the hypothalamus to the pituitary gland that regulates testosterone production in the testes, which leads to decreased male hormones. You need to get the right amount of calories to support testosterone increase and muscle growth without adding body fat.

Protein

Surprised? While many health experts preach the importance of protein, make no mistake, it is crucial to get sufficient amounts, when you want to increase your testosterone production. Research shows that eating more protein than carbohydrates may reduce the T-hormone level, as well as increases cortisol level.

Polyunsaturated Fat

I have mentioned earlier that you need to consume a significant amount of fat to boost testosterone production. However, you should not overload your body with polyunsaturated fats since they lower T-hormone level.

Too Much Caffeine

Too many cups of Joe increases cortisol level, which by now you know too well, decreases the production of the male hormone. Moreover, caffeinated drinks hurt your sleeping schedule, which also reduces testosterone level since the body cannot secrete T-hormone efficiently and regulate cortisol level.

TOO MUCH ALCOHOLIC DRINK

Avoid hitting the bottle hard. Alcohol affects the parts of the hypothalamic-pituitary-gonadal (HPG) axis, an endocrine hormones and glands system involved in testosterone production. Alcohol consumption lowers the T-hormone level in various ways.

- One of the ingredients used to make beer, the hops, are estrogenic, which converts male sex hormone T into female sex hormone estrogen.

- Ethanol metabolism lowers the amount of a particular coenzyme that is vital in the production of androgens, including testosterone.

- Alcohol stimulates endorphin production, which negatively affects T synthesis.

- Drinking alcoholic beverages damage cells of the testes, the primary producer of testosterone.

- The combination of cortisol and alcohol destroys circulating testosterone.

EXPOSURE TO T-LOWERING CHEMICALS

The common chemicals found in your home may be causing damaging effects to your testosterone level. These compound are what endocrinologists call "endocrine disruptors," which interfere with your hormone system, causing various problems like learning disabilities and weight gain.

Xenoestrogens

You need to be wary of this particular endocrine disruptor. Xenoestrogens are chemicals that imitate estrogen in the body. When your body is exposed to too much of estrogen-imitating chemical, the male hormone production drops significantly.

Some endocrinologists suggest that xenoestrogens are the reason why men today have lower T level than in the past decade. Moreover, doctors claim that expectant mothers should avoid these chemicals during pregnancy to prevent hypospadias, a congenital disability in male babies in which the opening of the penis is on the underside and not the tip.

Foods that Kill Testosterone

Soy-Based Food

Cereals, baked goods, snacks, salad, dressings, mayonnaise, all the processed food, commercial milk, cheeses, and yogurts, and sugar crush your testosterone. These foods are in one way or another contaminated with soy, as well as hormones. However, that does not mean you should avoid dairy products. Just make sure you buy organic and those that come from sources where they do not inject their animals with estrogenic hormones.

Busting the Myth of Steroids and Drugs

The popularity of using steroid use, testosterone replacement therapy, and testosterone supplements to increase male hormone production is on the rise. Every man wants to become manlier fast! But do these solutions really work?

Fat Loss

In relation to body fat percentage, men with naturally higher testosterone level are leaner, even when there is a fluctuation in male hormone of about 100 to 200 ng/dL. However, studies show that fat mass rose when T level decreases more than 200 ng/dL, For example, when a man's average range drops from 600 to about 300 ng/dL, body fat rose to about 36 percent. Just increasing your testosterone is useful if you only want to get rid of excess body fat. But what about for those who want to be more bulky and robust?

Muscle Growth and Strength

Using drugs indeed raise testosterone levels dramatically and no one can argue the powerful fat-burning and muscle-building effects of steroids. But what most people do not know is that **increasing T-hormone level within the healthy range does not help muscle growth.**

Various research and studies reveal that raising your male **hormone through the roof with anabolic steroids and drugs do not result in shocking muscle gain.** The only way testosterone level is going to make a significant increase is muscle mass and strength, even when you do not add exercise into your regimen, is when the amount exceeds the highest natural range by around 20 to 30 percent, approximately 1,200 ng/dL. As we have mentioned earlier, excessive amounts of the ultimate male hormone cause various detrimental effects in the long run. You will be paying a high price for it – your health.

The bottom line, small fluctuations in your testosterone levels will not make any difference in your muscle mass and strength unless you go to both, either extraordinarily high or tremendously low. Moreover, various factors, including training history, genetics, workout programming, diet, etc. affect muscle growth and strength. Thus, just raising you T level with drugs and anabolic steroids is not enough to help you look manlier.

If you are increasing your ultimate male hormone for larger muscles, then you have to exercise and workout. You cannot achieve a muscular physique without breaking any sweat.

Key Takeaways:

- Your lifestyle and habits dramatically influence the production of the ultimate male hormone.

- The body makes almost all the T it needs for the day during sleeping, so insufficient sleep kills your manliness.

- Men who sleep less than 5 hours every week are less manly.

- Sleep also regulates the stress hormone, cortisol, that the body releases throughout the day to meet the challenges and demands.

- High cortisol level significantly lowers T production.

- Stress elevates cortisol level, which kills your testosterone.

- Fat is a vital source of cholesterol, the building blocks of testosterone. Consuming less than 20 percent of calories from fat sabotages your man hormones.

- Eating more protein than carbohydrates may reduce the T-hormone level, as well as increases cortisol level.

- Polyunsaturated fat lowers the ultimate male hormone.

- Too much caffeine disrupts your sleep, as well as increases cortisol level, enemies of your testosterone.

- Alcohol affects the parts of the hypothalamic-pituitary-gonadal (HPG) axis, an endocrine hormones and glands system involved in testosterone production.

- Alcoholic drinks contain estrogenic ingredients converts male sex hormone T into female sex hormone estrogen.

- These chemical are what endocrinologists call "endocrine disruptors," which interfere with your hormone system. Xenoestrogens are chemicals that imitate estrogen in the body. When your body is exposed to too much of estrogen-imitating chemical, the male hormone production drops significantly.

- Soy-based food kills the ultimate male hormone.

- When your average T range drops than 200 ng/dL, your body fat rises to about 36 percent.

- Synthetic steroid to increase your testosterone is sufficient if you only want to get rid of excess body fat, but it will not help you build and strengthen muscles.

- Merely increasing T-hormone level within the healthy range using synthetic steroids and drugs do not help muscle growth, unless the amount exceeds the highest natural range by around 20 to 30 percent, roughly 1,200 ng/dL, which has cause various detrimental effects in the long run.

- Merely raising you T level with drugs and anabolic steroids will not help you look manlier since various factors, including training history, genetics, workout programming, diet, etc. affect muscle growth and strength.

Chapter 5 – How to boost your testosterone naturally

Boost your testosterone production without resorting to drug and anabolic steroid use is possible. However, the devil is in the details. Here what you need to do precisely to increase your male hormone efficiently.

Get Enough Rest

Sleeping only 3 to 5 hours at night is a testosterone killer! Sleep for about 8 to 9 hours every night as much as possible. Go to bed early, cutting the time that you would have wasted surfing the internet mindlessly.

Moreover, to improve the quality of your sleep, do the following:

- Reduce your exposure to blue light.
- Reduce your caffeine consumption.
- Take warm showers before going to bed.

Relax

Stress increases the levels of cortisol in your body. High levels of this stress hormone have the reverse effect on your testosterone level. Various studies show the there is a decrease in free T-hormone amount in the blood when the cortisol level is high. Here are some ways that you can combat stress.

- Relaxation exercises and meditation are very effective at reducing cortisol and raising T-hormone

- Walking in nature, such as hiking, forest walking, significantly lowers cortisol levels in many people.

- Adaptogenic herbs, such as Shilajit, Ashwagandha, Rhodiola Rosea, etc., lowers cortisol and increase testosterone simultaneously by helping the adrenal system regulate hormones.

- Vitamin C reduces cortisol secretion during stress, as well as relieves the damaging effects of stress hormones.

- Low-intensity exercises relieve stress. Avoid high-intensity physical exertions since they elevate cortisol level.

- Get sufficient amount of carbohydrates. A low-carb diet during stress increases cortisol secretion since the body is not getting enough glucose, its primary source of energy. Moreover, when you are not consuming the right amount of carbs, stresses the body more due to a low source of fuel.

Consume More Monounsaturated and Unsaturated fat

Avoid polyunsaturated fats (PUFAs), which are mostly in plant-based foods and oils. You should avoid salmon and other fatty fish since they are high in omega-3 fatty acids, which are the most potent form of polyunsaturated fats.

PUFAs are liquid at room temperatures, such as margarine, fish oil, cottonseed oil, sunflower seed oil, canola oil, and soybean oil. Increased intake of these oils suppresses male hormone production. Transfat also decreases testosterone level, so you also need to avoid food with this fat.

Monounsaturated Fat (MUFAs)

These types of fats are also liquid at room temperatures, such as extra-virgin olive oil and argan oil. Other sources of MUFAs are avocado, nuts, and seeds.

Saturated fatty-acids (SFAs)

These types of fats are hard at room temperatures, such as those found in dairy products, red meat, palm oil, cacao butter, lard, coconut oi, and butter.

MUFAs and SFAs Increases Testosterone Level

Research shows that T level plummets when a person is consuming a low-fat diet. Men who eat a low-fat diet and high in PUFAs tend to have significantly lower male hormones.

How Much Fat Should I Consume?

Will I have higher testosterone level if I eat more fat? NO. You also have to consume sufficient amount of carbohydrates and protein. The optimal dietary fat intake for efficient male hormone production is between 25 to 40 percent of your daily calorie requirement.

If you can reduce your PUFA intake, then you can lower your fat consumption to 25 percent and still keep your testosterone level high. However, if you consume polyunsaturated fat, it is better to eat between 30 to 40 percent of your total calorie requirement from fat.

It is vital that you do not exceed 40 percent since you have to make room for protein and carbohydrates.

Moreover, consuming sufficient amounts of fat helps you recover from physical exertion. Low fat consumption compromises your recovery from exercise, even moderate intensity.

Consume the Right Amount of Carbohydrate and Protein

Let's move from the correct amount of fat. The next step is to get the right amount of protein and carbohydrate.

How Much Should I Eat?

Consume at least 2 grams of carbohydrates and no more and no less than 1 gram of protein per 1 pound of your body weight each day, keeping the ratio of carbs and protein at 2:1.

Make sure that you get your protein from animal sources since a vegan causes low T-hormone level. Also, make sure get enough refined carbs since a high-fiber tend to reduce testosterone. Of course, choose the healthy kind of refined carbs, such as white rice and cream of wheat. Always avoid processed food.

REDUCE CAFFEINE INTAKE

You do not have to eliminate a cup of Joe in your diet. In fact, you can limit yourself to 200 milligrams of caffeine, about 2 cups of coffee a day. Studies show that caffeine helps boost testosterone level.

However, do not exceed the recommended daily amount. Too much coffee increases the level of cortisol in your body, which kills the male hormone.

Reduce Alcohol Consumption

A moderate amount, about 1 ½ glasses of red wine, lower T by 7 percent. Although too much alcohol kills testosterone, a low dosage, approximately 0.5 grams per kilogram of alcohol or 10% weight per volume, actually increase T-hormone slightly.

However, a study reports that 1 gram per kilogram alcohol, about a ½ glass of vodka for most males, taken after workout increased the male hormone by 100 percent. But that doesn't mean you should drink alcohol before working out because one study revealed that working out with a hangover or drunk increase the lowering effects of alcohol significantly.

Avoid Xenoestrogens

These chemicals are abundant. Avoid products that contain xenoestrogens as much as you possibly can, including the following:

- Plastic containers that contain phthalates, as well as foods that are stored or heated food in plastic containers. Keep your food in glassware.

- Gasoline and pesticides – wash your hands if you after exposure to them.

- Bisphenol A (BPA) containing products, like plastics used in water bottles, and products coated with epoxy resins, such as drink and food cans.

Aside from avoiding the products mentioned above, you should also do the following:

- Choose organic food. As mentioned, pesticides contain xenoestrogens. If your budget does not allow you to afford organic, always wash your vegetables and fruits thoroughly before eating. Also, find meat and animal products from animals that have not been treated with hormones.

- Use organic bath products. Most grooming products today, about 75 percent, contain parabens, a type of xenoestrogen. Use paraben-free, natural products.

HIT THE GYM

Exercise helps boost the male hormone in two ways. First, it helps reduce body fat and raise muscle mass. As mentioned earlier, fat converts testosterone to estrogen, so the less fat you have, the higher your T-hormone.

Second, the specific types of exercise below actually stimulate the body to secrete more testosterone.

Lift Weights

You have to start lifting –heavy weights! Here is the best weightlifting routine to maximize the production of your male hormone.

- Make compound lifts, such as shoulder press, deadlift, bench press, and squats, your main lifts. Exercising the large muscle groups increase T-hormone.

- Use a workout volume following the sets x reps x weight formula. Studies suggest higher volume result in higher testosterone production.

- Do not push yourself to failure for all your sets. It is okay to do it on your very last set.

- Rest for more than 1 minute and less than 2 minutes between your sets.

High-Intensity Interval Training (HIIT)

Studies show that HIIT workouts or repeated burst of intense exercises followed by a less-intense period for recovery boosts the male hormone production, as well as increase fat metabolism, muscle strength, and improve athletic conditioning.

There are various HIIT workouts, but the simplest one is a simple wind sprint routine. For example, you can sprint for 20 yards and rest for about 1 minute, doing 20 sets of sprint and rest.

Do Not Overtrain!

As important as doing the right exercises, giving your body the chance to rest and recuperate is just as important. Exercising until exhaustion significantly reduces the male hormone. As mentioned earlier, workouts release cortisol levels, which lowers testosterone level.

Rest for at least 2 days every week – do not do any intense workout during these days. However, the number of rest days will depend on the intensity of your exercise. Give yourself more rest time as needed.

During your rest days, you can go on a light hike or walk, which is also a great way to relieve stress.

HIT THE SACK

You know that testosterone increases sex drive. But the most enjoyable way to boost testosterone level is regular sexual activity; this works for both men and women. In females, the T-hormone is what makes them desire penetration. A study shows that males and females have higher T level after sexual activity.

So the rumors about having too much sex, as well as masturbation, drains testosterone is simply incorrect. However, sex raises the male hormone by 72 percent while masturbation only increases the amount by 11 percent.

Moreover, higher T level also makes you want to have more sex, which brings you to a positive loop.

TAKE COLD SHOWERS

Many men view that keeping the balls cold as a simple myth. However, various studies in humans and animals show that the testes perform better when they are around 87 to 96 degrees Fahrenheit. Higher temperatures affect spermatogenesis, DNA synthesis, and testosterone production negatively.

Moreover, other research shows that sperm motility, quality, and volume are higher during cold months. The same hormones that are responsible spermatogenesis, luteinizing hormone (LH) and follicle-stimulating hormone (FSH), are also the ones responsible for testosterone synthesis, so a link exists.

So aside from taking cold showers daily, you might want to wear loose boxer shorts and sleep naked to keep your balls cool.

Aside from keeping the balls cool, taking a cold shower also improves the quality of your sleep, which is also vital in testosterone production since the body produces the male hormone it needs for the day while you are sleeping.

BULK UP WITH THESE

As vital as avoiding testosterone killers, knowing what to put in your body is also significant to become manlier. Here are the right food and supplements that will optimize our body's ability to produce testosterone.

30 Foods that Boost testosterone Levels

1. Grapes

Chinese researchers revealed that 500 milligrams of grapes, about 5 to 10 grams of grape skin, increase the male hormone level, as well as improve the sperms' swimming ability. The resveratrol in the grape skin makes you manlier.

2. Tuna

One can of tuna supplies your body with 100 percent of your recommended daily allowance of vitamin D, which boosts T-hormone by up to 90 percent.

3. Pomegranate

Research shows that a glass of pomegranate juice improves sexual drive by up to 47 percent.

4. Venison

Going on a meat-free diet lowers T level by 14 percent. However, a diet rich in saturated fat, found in lamb and beef, can also reduce testosterone. Go for the middle ground, venison.

5. Garlic

Allicin, a compound in garlic reduces cortisol, a stress hormone, thus, increasing testosterone level. Each clove is more potent when taken raw than cooked.

6. Honey

Boron, a trace mineral found in honey is significant to the body's use of testosterone, estrogen, and vitamin D, as well as boosts magnesium, another mineral vital to T-hormone production. The sweet liquid is also rich in nitric oxide, which opens the blood vessels for better erectile function.

7. Milk

The amino acids in milk increase anabolic hormone production, which trims fat and build muscles.

8. Eggs

The cholesterol found in egg yolks stimulates T production. They also contain omega-3 fatty acids, vitamin D, and saturated fat, which are all critical for the male hormone production.

9. Cabbage

The cruciferous vegetable is rich in indole-3-carbinol that flushes out estrogen or the female hormone. Research shows that consuming 500 grams for 7 days flushes out half of men's estrogen in men, making T-hormone production more efficient.

10. Asparagus

The spears are aphrodisiac. They contain vitamin E, potassium, and folic acid, which are all vital for T production.

11. Bananas

The fruit helps increase testosterone level through the enzyme bromelain. They are also an excellent source of slow-releasing energy, perfect for a passionate night.

12. Watermelon

The refreshing fruit contains citrulline, an amino acid that the body converts into arginine, which increases blood flow.

13. Ginseng

Research in 2002 revealed that Korean red ginseng Korean red ginseng helps improve erectile dysfunction by up to 60 percent.

14. Almonds

A handful of these nuts is a rich source of zinc, which boosts testosterone and enhances libido. The mineral increases the sex drive of both males and females. S

15. Oysters

The seafood delight is the most abundant source of zinc.

16. Porridge Oats

Not only do these contain zinc, but they also contain L-arganine and high in B vitamins, which boost sexual performance.

17. Citrus Fruits

These fruits lower the amount of cortisol in the body, increasing testosterone. They also contain vitamin A, which is essential in T production and also help reduce the female hormone estrogen.

18. Spinach

The leafy green lowers estrogen amount. They are also rich in vitamin C, E, and magnesium, which are all testosterone building blocks.

19. Wild Salmon

Aside from high amounts of omega-3 fatty acids, vitamin B, and magnesium, this fish lower sex hormone binding globulin (SHBG) level, which renders testosterone inactive. Thus, you have more free or active T-hormone.

20. Avocado

As mentioned earlier, men need to consume healthy amounts of monounsaturated fat like vegetable oils and nuts. Avocadoes are a rich source of MUFAs. These fats also lower LDL cholesterol or bad cholesterol, aside from boosting the male hormone level.

21. Tuna

If you do not get enough sunshine, then eat more tuna. They are rich in vitamin D that boosts testosterone production by up to 90 percent. The sunshine vitamin is also vital for keeping your sperm count and sperm quality high.

22. Meat

As mentioned earlier, going on a meat-free diet kills your testosterone. However, you should only consume the right amount. Eating high amounts of saturated fat lowers T-hormone as well. Grass-fed beef and bison meat are great options. A reminder, choose organic as much as possible to avoid estrogenic hormones injected in meat.

23. Shrimp

Consuming this seafood is a sure way to increase your vitamin D, which is linked to higher amounts of testosterone. Moreover, males and females with high levels of this vitamin in their blood have stronger lower and upper body muscle strength. You can also get the sunshine vitamin in mackerel, sardines, salmon, free-range eggs, and herring.

24. Pumpkin Seeds

Research shows that low zinc is linked to low testosterone level. These seeds are an excellent source of the mineral, which is involved in various enzymatic reactions, including the production of the male hormone. You can also get more of this nutrient from lentils, cashews, sesame seeds, wheat germ, steak, chicken, turkey, and crab.

25. Coconut and Olive Oil

Coconut oil is a rich source of saturated fat. You can get up to 10 percent of your calories from this fat without increasing your risk of heart problems. Chocolate, red palm oil, lamb, steak, full-fat dairy, and butter are also excellent sources of saturated fatty acids.

This fat is also an excellent source of MCT oil, an excellent source of energy that helps increase metabolic rate, boost thyroid hormones, and enhance cognitive performance.

As mentioned earlier, healthy amounts of monounsaturated fat make you manlier and long-lasting virility. A study revealed that 2 weeks of olive oil as the primary dietary fat source increase T level up to 17 percent.

Moreover, this healthy oil is an excellent source of antioxidant and has anti-inflammatory properties. Add 1 to 2 tablespoons of this fat to your daily salad.

26. Wheat Bran

The fiber-rich bran is an excellent source of magnesium. Research shows that higher amount of this mineral increases T level, especially when you do HIIT exercises. You can add wheat bran to your protein shakes, pancake batter, and oatmeal. You can also increase your magnesium from beans, butter, peanut butter, sunflower seeds, oat bran, whole grains, almonds, and cocoa powder.

27. Ricotta Cheese

The best source of whey protein is this dairy product. Whey protein is rich in amino acids, which decreases cortisol level in the body, especially during after recovery from intense training. Add kefir, yogurt, milk, and whey protein powder in your diet to get more amino acids.

28. Strawberries

The best source of vitamin C, strawberries is an excellent source of potent antioxidant, which lowers cortisol level, especially after hard workouts.

29. Celery

The scent alone can boost T level! They contain androstenone and androstenol, two important plant sterols. The names alone indicate that they have a significant effect on the production and action of androgens.

They are also an excellent source of flavonoids, some of which are anti-estrogenic agents like luteolin and some are natural T-hormone boosters, like apigenin.

30. Fava Beans

The beans contain L-dopa, which increases dopamine levels in the brain, increasing T level. L-dopa also boosts the human growth hormone, which builds more muscle.

31. Broccoli

They contain diindolemethyl (DIM), a potent anti-estrogen compound. DIM improves estrogen metabolism, allowing higher production of testosterone.

Other foods that also help boost testosterone production include the following:

- Potatoes. All kinds are an excellent source of gluten-free carbohydrates.
- Macadamia nuts
- Beef gelatin
- Brazil nuts
- Raisins
- Parsley
- Ginger
- Raw cacao products
- Real salt
- Argan oil

- White button mushrooms
- Baking soda
- Grass-fed beef jerky
- Organic minced meat
- Blue cheese
- 'Dark Berries, such as acai berries, blackberries, and blueberries
- Sorghum
- Onion

Supplements that Aid Testosterone Production

If you are on a loose budget, you can boost your vitamins and minerals requirement by taking supplements. Here are some nutritional boosters that are proven to produce significant positive effects on testosterone level.

Vitamin D3

D3 not a vitamin, but a hormone that provides significant health benefits to the body and vital for testosterone production. It's the precursor to vitamin D production.

The body cannot create the sunshine vitamin naturally. During winter months and when you are spending less time outdoors, you are prone to vitamin D deficiency, which contributes to low T-hormone level.

Studies show that taking 3332 IU of vitamin D3 for 1 year increases testosterone level up to 25.2 percent. If you are dark skinned, you may need to intake a higher dosage, about 4000 IU.

Moreover, you can also boost your vitamin D via UV light exposure s to stimulate the male hormone.

Zinc

Zinc deficiency is not common. Research shows that 30 milligrams of zinc daily increases levels of active testosterone in the body of men with hypogonadism. If you are a healthy man 19 years old and above, you only need to take 11 milligrams daily, or you may not need to if you are consuming your recommended daily amount.

Not that you should never take more than the recommended dosage or more than 40 milligrams daily since too much of this mineral can lead to toxicity with symptoms of abdominal cramps, diarrhea, vomiting, headaches, and nausea.

Magnesium

Deficiency of this mineral is more common than zinc. The recommended daily dosage of this mineral is 420 milligram daily for adult males. To enhance your testosterone production, take about 750 milligrams daily for 1 week and see how it goes.

Key Takeaways:

- Rest for 8 to 9 hours every night to help your body regulate cortisol level and produce testosterone efficiently during your sleep. Waking up with a "morning wood" is a sure sign that you are manlier than finding it limp.

- Find ways to combat stress and reduce cortisol production.

- Men who consume a diet low in fat and high in polyunsaturated fat (PUFAs) tend to have significantly lower male hormones. Consume more monounsaturated Fat (MUFAs) and saturated fatty acids (SFAs).

- Get 25 to 40 percent of your daily calorie requirement from MUFAs and SFAs.

- You can consume 25 percent of your daily calorie requirement from fat when you reduce your PUFA intake.

- If you consume polyunsaturated fat, it is better to eat between 30 to 40 percent of your total calorie requirement from fat.

- Do not exceed 40 percent of your daily calorie requirement from fat since you have to make room for protein and carbohydrates.

- The effective ratio of carbohydrates and protein for boosting testosterone is 2:1. Consume at least 2 grams of carbs and no more and no less than 1 gram of protein per 1 pound of your body weight each day.

- Caffeine helps boost testosterone level, but limit your intake 200 milligrams of caffeine, about 2 cups of coffee a day. Any more than that will kill your manliness.

- About 0.5 grams per kilogram of alcohol or 10% weight per volume, actually increase T-hormone slightly. Higher dosage sabotages your T.

- One gram per kilogram alcohol, about 1/2 glass of vodka for most males, taken after workout increased the male hormone by 100 percent. However, do not do any exercise with a hangover or drunk. You will kill your testosterone.

- Avoid products with xenoestrogens as, such as plastic containers, gasoline, pesticides, and bisphenol A (BPA) containing products, like the plastic used in water bottles, and products coated with epoxy resins, such as drink and food cans.

- Choose organic food and use organic products.

- The best workout to boost your testosterone levels are weights and high-intensity interval training (HIIT)

- Overtraining kills your hormone since it does not give your body the chance to recuperate and regulate cortisol level secreted during a workout. Giving your body enough time to rest is vital.

- Sex raises the male hormone by 72 percent while masturbation only increases the amount by 11 percent. Moreover, higher T level also makes you want to have more sex, which brings you to a positive loop.

- Taking a bath helps bolster your manliness. The testes perform better when they are around 87 to 96 degrees Fahrenheit. Higher temperatures affect spermatogenesis, DNA synthesis, and testosterone production negatively.

- Cold bath improves the quality of your sleep, vital in testosterone production since the body produces the male hormone it needs for the day while you are sleeping.

- Knowing what to put in your body is also significant to become manlier. The right food and supplements will optimize our body's ability to produce testosterone.

Final Words

Thank you again for purchasing this book! I really hope this book is able to help you.

The next step is for you to **join our email newsletter** to receive updates on any upcoming new book releases or promotions. You can sign-up for free and as a bonus, you will also receive our "*7 Fitness Mistakes You Don't Know You're Making*" book! This bonus book breaks down many of the most common fitness mistakes and will demystify many of the complexities and science of getting into shape. Having all this fitness knowledge and science organized into an actionable step-by-step book will help you get started in the right direction in your fitness journey! To join our free email newsletter and grab your free book, please visit the link and signup: **www.hmwpublishing.com/gift**

Finally, if you enjoyed this book, then I would like to ask you for a favour, would you be kind enough to leave a review for this book? It would be greatly appreciated!

Thank you and good luck in your journey!

About the Co-Author

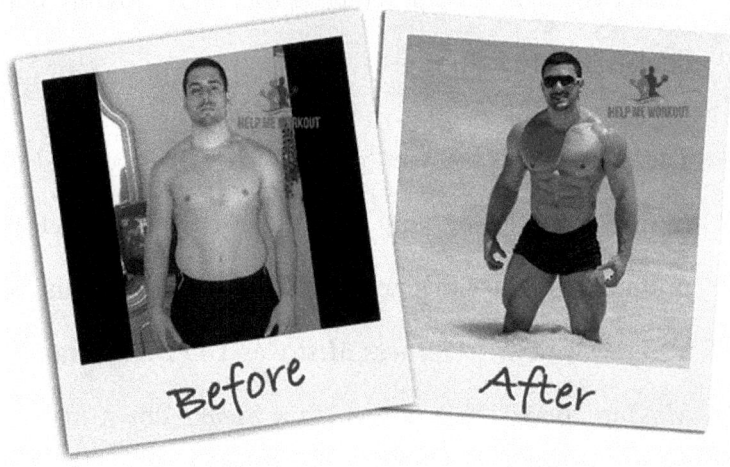

My name is George Kaplo; I'm a certified personal trainer from Montreal, Canada. I'll start off by saying I'm not the biggest guy you will ever meet and this has never really been my goal. In fact, I started working out to overcome my biggest insecurity when I was younger, which was my self-confidence. This was due to my height measuring only 5 foot 5 inches (168cm), it pushed me down to attempt anything I ever wanted to achieve in life. You may be going through some challenges right now, or you may simply want to get fit, and I can certainly relate.

For me personally, I was always kind of interested in the

health & fitness world and wanted to gain some muscle due to the numerous bullying in my teenage years about my height and my overweight body. I figured I couldn't do anything about my height, but I sure can do something about how my body looked like. This was the beginning of my transformation journey. I had no idea where to start, but I just got started. I felt worried and afraid at times that other people would make fun of me for doing the exercises the wrong way. I always wished I had a friend that was next to me who was knowledgeable enough to help me get started and "show me the ropes."

After a lot of work, studying and countless trial and errors. Some people began to notice how I was getting more fit and how I was starting to form a keen interest in the topic. This led many friends and new faces to come to me and ask me for fitness advice. At first, it seemed odd when people asked me to help them get in shape. But what kept me going is when they started to see changes in their own body and told me it's the first time that they saw real results! From there, more people kept coming to me, and it made me realize after so much reading and studying in this field that it did help me but it also allowed me to help others. I'm now a fully certified personal trainer and have trained numerous clients to date who have achieved amazing results.

Today, my brother Alex Kaplo (also a Certified Personal Trainer) and I own & operate this publishing venture, where we bring passionate and expert authors to write about health and fitness topics. We also run an online fitness website "HelpMeWorkout.com" and I would love to connect with by inviting you to visit the website on the following page and signing up to our e-mail newsletter (you will even get a free book).

Last but not least, if you are in the position I was once in and you want some guidance, don't hesitate and ask... I'll be there to help you out!

Your friend and coach,

George Kaplo
Certified Personal Trainer

Get another book for Free

I want to thank you for purchasing this book and offer you another book (just as long and valuable as this book), "Health & Fitness Mistakes You Don't Know You're Making", completely free.

Visit the link below to signup and receive it:

www.hmwpublishing.com/gift

In this book, I will break down the most common health & fitness mistakes, you are probably committing right now, and I will reveal how you can easily get in the best shape of your life!

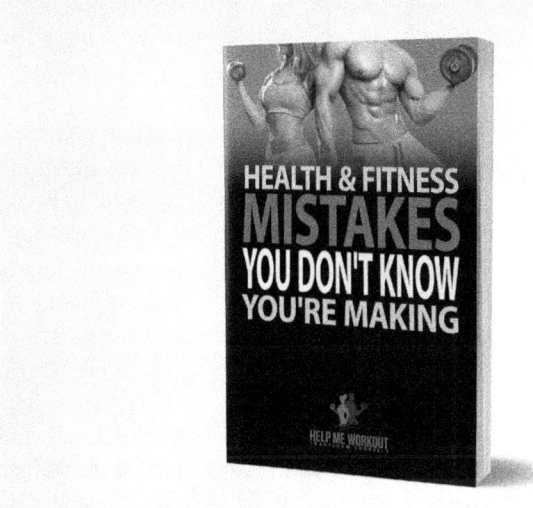

In addition to this valuable gift, you will also have an opportunity to get our new books for free, enter giveaways, and receive other valuable emails from me. Again, visit the link to sign up:

www.hmwpublishing.com/gift

Copyright 2017 by HMW Publishing - All Rights Reserved.

This document by HMW Publishing owned by the A&G Direct Inc company, is geared towards providing exact and reliable information in regards to the topic and issue covered. The publication is sold with the idea that the publisher is not required to render accounting, officially permitted, or otherwise, qualified services. If advice is necessary, legal or professional, a practiced individual in the profession should be ordered.

From a Declaration of Principles which was accepted and approved equally by a Committee of the American Bar Association and a Committee of Publishers and Associations.

In no way is it legal to reproduce, duplicate, or transmit any part of this document in either electronic means or in printed format. Recording of this publication is strictly prohibited, and any storage of this document is not allowed unless with written permission from the publisher. All rights reserved.

The information provided herein is stated to be truthful and consistent, in that any liability, in terms of inattention or otherwise, by any usage or abuse of any policies, processes, or directions contained within is the solitary and utter responsibility of the recipient reader. Under no circumstances will any legal responsibility or blame be held against the publisher for any reparation, damages, or monetary loss due to the information herein, either directly or indirectly.

The information herein is offered for informational purposes solely, and is universal as so. The presentation of the information is without contract or any type of guarantee assurance.

The trademarks that are used are without any consent, and the publication of the trademark is without permission or backing by the trademark owner. All trademarks and brands within this book are for clarifying purposes only and are the owned by the owners themselves, not affiliated with this document.

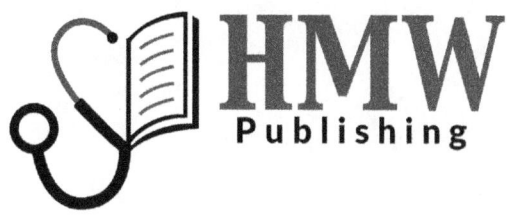

For more great books visit:

HMWPublishing.com

www.ingramcontent.com/pod-product-compliance
Lightning Source LLC
Chambersburg PA
CBHW071113030426
42336CB00013BA/2061